Healing Salve

Homemade Recipes Of Herbal Balms And Salves

Book Description

Master solution and salve making and create your own products only just how you like them. Save money at the same time. What's more, making these types of products is like soap and candle making.

Get these tips about assembling balms and salves sell or to use.

Tip 1 - body butters and Salves, balms are all made about the same way. Containers usually are different. Other than that, the principle difference in only in the amounts of the resources used to make-up the products.

Tip 2 - Salves and balms are actually just combinations of a wax and butters or oils. That simple mixture is all it will take to make a salve item. Using more waxes usually gets you a product that is tougher. Applying less wax results and more oils in a thing that is softer.

Tip 3 - Combining essential oils into the products can be a way to get a particular perfume to the mixture and a way to provide some herbal substance to the product also. The practitioner of aromatherapy recognizes a salve being a service for the primary oil.

Tip 4 - tweak recipes to allow for changes in weather, heat mainly If you create your own balms. It is good to possess a harder merchandise, that is not as likely to melt and work, because the weather gets really warm. Conversely, in cold places or in the cool part of the season, a softer solution is nicer to use.

Tip 5 - People like to buy these types of natural products. That is so partly while there is a whole lot of interest in preventing artificial substances around the skin.

Which means individuals are getting far from many lotions. These types of products are quite similar as balms, but without all of the chemicals.

Of course a limitless variety of variations to the salves design are possible. Vary the ingredients in these mixes and vary the ratios and get all types of benefits. This makes assembling these types of resources really an interesting hobby.

Additionally, it makes solution and salve making a probable gains generator too.

Introduction

There is little doubt that interest in natural healing techniques are at an all-time high. More and more, individuals are looking for ways to soothe their health with natural remedies which might be truly effective. It is important to note below that you should never self-diagnose. Speak with your doctor and ensure that you do not have significant underlying problems that need to be handled by a doctor.

One of the most flexible products for your skin will be the salve. There is a salve an ointment that is built with some kind of wax and some sort of oil. It's semi-soft, and blends easily to the skin. With respect to the oil and the wax, it remains on the top or may soak readily to the skin. Salves can lend water to your skin along with become a protective barrier.

HEALING SALVE

This menu can be a simple one which you'll employ over and once again. The ingredients are:

-One and one half ounce of beeswax

-16 Ounces of oil

To prepare, serve 16 ounces of sweet almond oil into the top container of a double boiler. Change heat to gradually and low add approximately one and one-half ounces of beeswax. You can acquire beeswax from many places. Just perform a search on your favorite search engine for brown beeswax.

When the beeswax and service oil are combined together, you can include natural essential oils chosen for their healing properties. Like, if you need to use your salve to relieve pains and muscle cramps, placed around 15 drops of pure Camphor essential oil in the mix. Camphor can be a natural anesthetic, and is effective for achy and sore muscles. Eliminate and wax from the warmth before adding your essential oils.

Chapter 1 – THE BASICS OF MAKING BALMS AND SALVES

Lotions and salves are simply the same thing, the only difference being in the inclusion of crucial oils. Salves usually include herbal oil and fat carrier oil. A solution contains the same things with the addition of essential oils. Because of how surprisingly herbs and essential oils go together, ointments are usually made by me at our house because oils and herbs each minister in other ways and they work together to carry more all over benefits.

To produce a balm or salve all you need is the following:

An herb infused oil with your desired herbs

Beeswax

Tins or jars

Essential oils if desired

Choosing Your Herbs:

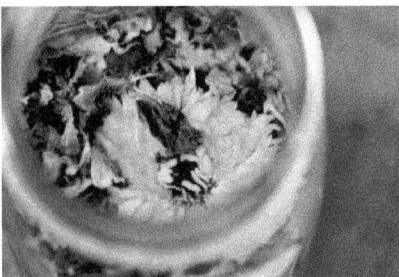

-you need to begin by choosing your herbs and making your herbal oil. You need to make certain that you review to ensure that you can safely handle each issue each ideal supplement to ensure of contraindications, its safety and employs.

-Don't feel overwhelmed by selecting the herbs you will use for your ointments! You don't have to have 20 herbs and a degree to use them. Select 3-5 herbs that you feel whenever they may interfere with any drugs and analyze them enough to know contraindications, properties, and their security and would be the most beneficial to what you're addressing you could be taking.

To make the herbal oil:

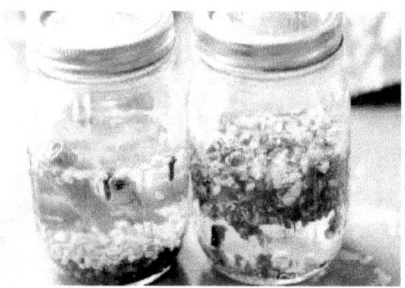

-Once you've chosen your herbs you need to pick a carrier oil. For ointments and salves I know like to stay with coconut oil, occasionally adding in some olive oil also. I love the coconut oil for its useful properties and also for how solid it is. Olive oil also offers some wonderful benefits for the skin and so I occasionally utilize a mixture with regards to the lotion I'm making.

-You can then determine the measurement of jar you wish to make based around the amount of product you want to have. I usually produce a pint sized container of oil as this usually equals about 2 large and 2 small jars of lotion which is plenty to hold over us for a little while. I also utilize a canning jar such that it is created to stand-up to the warmth of the crock pot.

-Fill your canning jar about 1/3 to 1/2 full of your desired herbs. Calculate out each herb based how you chose your herbs. I often employ more of my key plant than whatever else and then add smaller portions of the other herbs. Sometimes I use similar portions of each plant also. For my muscle balm I used more ginger than anything, and then the little less rose and arnica topped off with a few cinnamon sticks.

-Now put into your container your ideal carrier oil filling the bottle to the underside of the wheel. You might want to give it a moment to settle and adding more while the herbs will quickly soak up some of the oil. When working with strong coconut oil I usually melt it in a little skillet about the range over low temperature just enough to liquefy it before putting into the jars.

—Now prepare your crockpot and place your lid about the container. Place a thickly folded kitchen towel to the bottom of your crockpot. This keeps the vessel off of the underside of the box which helps to prevent it from cracking. Place your bottle to the cloth in the crockpot. Now complete the crock pot with water completely up to the bottom of the jar rim.

- Set the lid on the crockpot and transform it to the "Keep Warm" environment. Some individuals put on the "low" location, but for my crockpot I realized this is not too cold as my oils came out with a slightly burned smell. You would like to heat the oil allowing it to become without really cooking the herbs infused with the herbal properties.

-Keep the vessel in the crockpot warming for 3 days. Regularly check the water level to make certain it isn't dropping and if it does just keep adding water to maintain at the desired level.

-Once the 3 days are complete you allow it to cool and may remove your jar from your crockpot. You want to buy to be great enough to manage, however, not so awesome that it begins to harden if it's coconut oil. You may strain off the herbs once it's great enough to handle. Make sure you squeeze out every fall of oil you could thus you don't miss from any of the amazing oil! Now you have your herb infused oil!

Chapter 2 – Formulating Salves Recipes - Tips

If you are looking for salve recipes keep in mind that even really simple ingredients can work perfectly when the proportions of the ingredients are because they must be. In the end, the best salves are actually just a combination of a few ingredients. To get the best results with salves read on for a few tips.

Tip 1 - View for petrolatum in salves. That is a crude oil derivative. Simply because individuals have been rubbing these products all over themselves for nearly one hundred years does not mean that is an excellent idea. Many think it is not just a good idea. Instead of adding inexpensive oil based content on yourself, look for vegetable oils instead in the salve ingredients. That is s plus to making salves yourself. You can fit in what you want to use.

Tip 2 - Adding wax to oils may be the way you can quickly get the proper consistency to the salve you assembled. Usually a formula you notice may be 1/3 beeswax, 1/3 shea butter and 1/3 almond oil for a lip balm like product. That is a little bit too hard for my taste. It takes a little change.

Tip 3 - Though there are a wide range of waxes one can use to get the hardness in salves. It is very difficult to beat beeswax. The bee made feel features a wonderful scent and a pleasing waxy feel as well. In addition, the wax continues to be reasonable priced compared to alternatives. Just a touch will make a big change in oils to change them into a very nice paste.

Tip 4 - One of the most common methods to use as essential oils added to the salve as herbs infused to the oil or salves can be as a company for herbal products, sometimes. However, the salve alone has positive properties as a skin product, perhaps with no herbs included, provided you select the appropriate base oils to build the salve. There are always a range of excellent choices readily available.

Tip 5 - assembling salves can be a fun activity. That's so because you can find many combinations of supplies you can put together. Changing ingredients and dimensions of ingredients makes it easy to completely alter the final solution of a salve building program.

The invisible edge of creating salves is the great selection of products that one can put together using about procedures and the same ingredients. Body butters, glazes, herbal salves, lip balms and other products are really all about the exact same except for amounts of the various components. What's more, these simple substances can simply change for lotions, that will be advisable.

Chapter 3 – Some Salve Recipes

Healing Salve

Healing Salve Ingredients

2 cups olive oil or almond oil

1/4 cup beeswax pastilles

1 tsp echinacea root

2 Tbsp dried comfrey leaf

2 Tbsp dried plantain leaf

Instructions

Impress the herbs into the olive oil. There are two ways to do this. You can either incorporate the herbs and the olive oil in a jar with an airtight lid and leave 3-4 days, shaking daily OR heat the herbs and olive oil over low/low heat in a double boiler for 3 hours until the oil is extremely natural.

Stress her herbs out of the oil by putting through a cheesecloth. Allow all of the oil drip out and then fit the herbs to get the remaining oil out.

Discard the herbs.

Heat the infused oil in a double boiler with the beeswax until melted and mixed.

Pour into glass containers, small tins or top chap tubes and use on attacks, stings, reductions, poison ivy, diaper rash or other injuries as needed.

Vapor Rub

Vapor Rub Ingredients

1/2 cup olive oil, coconut oil, or almond oil

2 level tablespoons of beeswax pastilles

20 drops of Eucalyptus Oil

20 drops Peppermint Oil

10 drops Rosemary Oil

10 drops clove or cinnamon oil

Instructions

Melt beeswax with oil of choice in a double boiler until just melted.

Include the essential oils

Stir until well mixed and put into some kind of jar with a top to store. As do little jars, small tins work nicely.

Use as needed to help reduce congestion and coughing.

Make Herbal Infused Oil

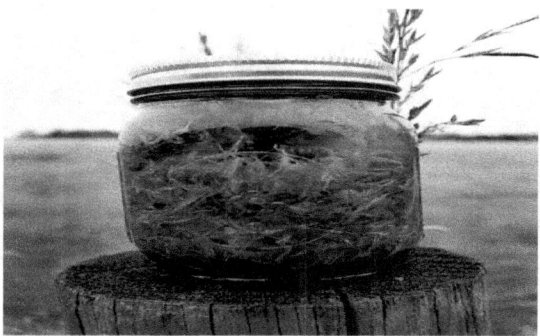

To make salve, first craft your herbal infused oil. This will take many weeks, but once completed, the others of the salve making process will simply take minutes! You can also purchase pre-infused herbal oils if you wish to miss out the process of infusing the oil or if required.

Solar Method: When making herbal infused oils, we like the solar infused method. Botanicals dried in to a sterilized and dry glass jar. Some herbalists coarsely crush or grind herbs first, while some leave delicate flowers whole and finely cut herbs. If desired, the jar may be covered with pack or a carrier so the oil is not subjected to direct sunlight. Move the jar normally as you remember, or a few times each day. You can add more oil in order that they are usually absorbed when the oil is absorbed by the herbs. Allow until the oil assumes smell and along with of the supplement, or to impress for 2-6 months. When the oil is ready, pressure using cheesecloth, and container into dry and sterilized amber bottles for storage. Make sure to squeeze from your herbs just as much oil as you can so that you do not waste any important oil! Organic oils could keep for around annually if stored correctly in a black and cool place. E Vitamin Gas may also be added to prolong the shelf life.

Quick Method: Another way to infuse oils, which will be sometimes necessary when herbal oils need to be produced in a touch, will be the quick method which utilizes heat. Much care needs to be used when making herbal oils in this way because you don't want to deep fry your herbs! Location herbs in crock pot, double boiler, or electronic yogurt maker, and cover with Extra Virgin Olive Oil causing at least an inch or two of oil above the erbs. Gently heat the herbs over very low temperature for 1-5 hours before oil takes on along with and odor of the herb. Some texts recommend heat 48-72 hours to the oil in a controlled heat of 100 degrees Fahrenheit. Switch off heat and allow to cool. Once that the oil is prepared, strain using cheesecloth, and container into sterilized amber bottles for storage and dry. Shop in a dark and neat spot, Vitamin Oil are often added to prolong the shelf life.

Beeswax for turning your infused oil in to a salve!

Part 2: Turn that Gas into Salve!

• 8 oz herbal infused oil(s) of your choice. Select a mix or one.

• 1 oz Beeswax

• Vitamin E Oil

• 10-20 drops essential oil of choice. Some essential oils popular are Rose and Tea tree.

• Glass Jars or Tin Containers

Place Herbal Infused Oils and Beeswax over a double boiler, and gently warm over low heat before the Beeswax melts. Remove from heat and incorporate the primary oil and E Vitamin Oil. Quickly put into prepared tins or glass containers and let to cool completely. Salves should be located in a very good spot where they'll remain semi solid and will not proceed to re-melt and re-solidify. If stored correctly, salves can last for 1- 3 years. Yields 8 oz.

Soothing Salve

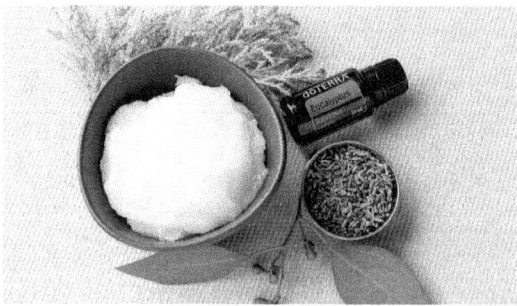

Ingredients:

1/2 cup grapeseed oil

1/2 cup almond oil

2 tablespoons beeswax

1/2 tablespoon vitamin E oil

5 drops Rose, Cypress, Melaleuca, Frankincense, and Eucalyptus essential oils

Directions:

Melt beeswax in double boiler.

Include grapeseed, almond once melted, and E Vitamin oil until melted.

Set aside for 2-3 minutes once blended.

Add essential oils and stir.

Fill in pot and allow to set for 2 hours.

To use, apply to skin or on chest.

Miracle Healing Salve

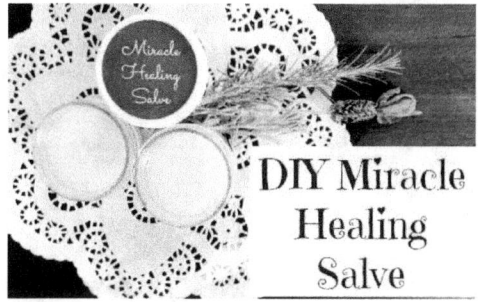

Ingredients:

1 Cup Coconut Oil

1 Cup Extra Virgin Olive Oil

5 Tbl. Organic Beeswax Pastilles

4 each – 4 ounce mason jars

1. Set of water to the range to simmer. As the water is heat, set the coconut oil, olive oil and beeswax pastilles in a heatproof bottle or measuring cup.

2. Set filled with the coconut oil, olive oil, and feel into the water till it melts, providing it a blend from time to time and keep it there. You'll need a slow, light

burn so take your time. It might take 20 or 15 minutes with respect to the temperature of the water bath.

3. Whilst the ingredients are melting, decrease your essential oils into each of the containers. Hint: I have discovered that it's easier to work with a glass medicine dropper compared to dropper that comes with the package of essential oil. That is recommended and a matter of personal choice.

4. Put into each of the smaller jars containing essential oils. There's no need to stir until you wish to because the oils may mixup independently.

5. Protect set them apart for up to 24 hours and the containers with cloth or a paper towel. It will take at least 12 hours to finish the firming process, although the salve will start to set within a few minutes.

HERB-INFUSED BALMS

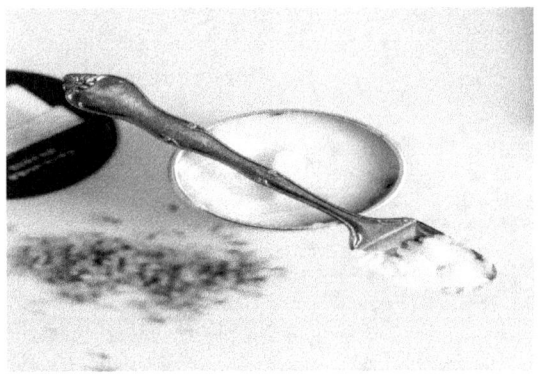

INGREDIENTS

Dried herbs

Carrier oil

Beeswax

Lidded containers

Essential oils

DIRECTIONS

Impress oils for 2-3 weeks in a tightly sealed box. Start again and you need to drop it if you discover mold growing.

Strain out the herbs

Mix oil and beeswax in saucepan or double broiler over low heat

When melted put into clear pots and incorporate essential oils if desired

Let salve cool and harden

Store in great, dry place in lidded box.

CUTICLE HEALING BALM

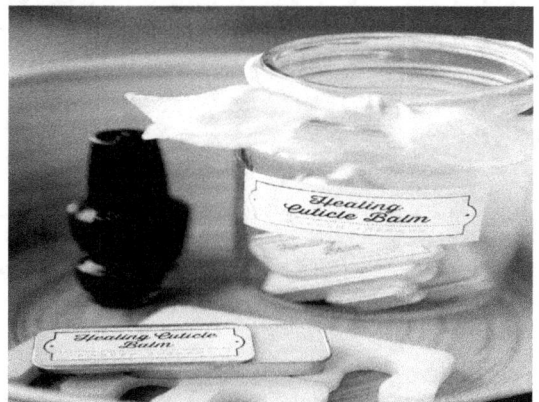

Ingredients:

• 1 tbsp coconut oil

• 1 tbsp hemp oil

• 1 tbsp sweet almond oil

• 1½ tbsp grated beeswax

• 1 tbsp mango butter

Equipment:

Boiler

• Small spatula or metal spoon

• 5 small metal tins or pots

Instructions:

1. Melt beeswax, oils and the apple butter in the double boiler.

2. Remove from heat, incorporate essential oils, and blend well.

3. Put into pots and leave untouched to set.

4. Add a custom rectangle label

BURN OINTMENT

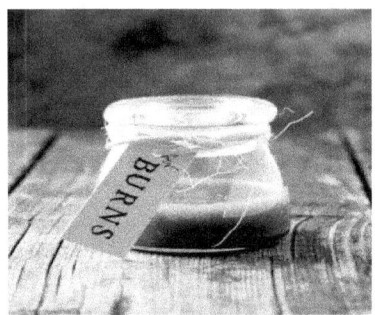

Ingredients:

1 part Calendula Flowers

1 part Comfrey Leaves

1 part Comfrey Root

1 part St John's Wort Flowers

1 part Olive Oil

Beeswax, grated

Place Saint and root John's wort flowers, comfrey leaves and the calendula flowers to the top section of a double boiler along with the olive oil, fill the underside with water, and carry it to a low boil.

Allow the oil simmer gently for 30-60 minutes, checking often to make sure the oil isn't overheating.

By getting it into the freezer for two or one minute to cool check a tiny amount for consistency. If it appears too hard, heat it again and add more oil. Reheat and add more beeswax, if it's too greasy.

While you've got the persistence you wish, move the ointment to clean glass jars. Located properly, creams last several months.

Natural Rosemary & Neem Oil Foot Salve Recipe

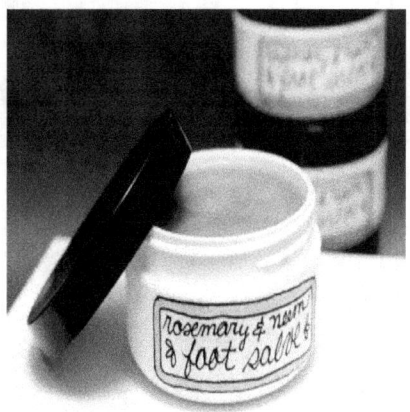

Ingredients:

4oz. pure lanolin

1 oz. raw beeswax

. Olive oil infused with comfrey leaves, plantain leaves & calendula blossoms

. shea butter

.25 oz. cocoa butter

1/2 teaspoon neem oil

1/4 teaspoon sea buckthorn oil

Instructions:

Begin by making your herb infused olive oil. Calendula flowers and comfrey leaves and position desired sum inside a mason jar to do this collect the plantain leaves. Cover with the container and tightly shut olive oil. Keep in an awesome, dark location turning occasionally for 4-6 weeks. To speed this process, position the mason jar of herbs and oil in a pot filled about 2/3 of just how full with water. Temperature around the oven on warm too low for 3-4 hours, then remove from heat and allow to cool. Strain the oil through cheesecloth back in your mason jar once you've implanted the olive oil with the botanicals.

You're prepared to make your foot salve after you have your infused oil.

Begin by weighing out the beeswax and cocoa butter using a digital scale and placing in to a double boiler and heat. Once these ingredients are 3/4 of the way melted, weigh out the shea butter and lanolin and include in to the double boiler.

Continue until all of the articles have melted entirely heating, then weigh out the infused herbal olive oil and mixture to the container. Remove from heat.

Using measuring spoons, measure the neem oil and sea buckthorn oil out and add to the salve base. Then with a brand new finished transfer pipette for each substance measure out and include the remaining ingredients. Mix well, then put into glass salve jars or tins and let to cool completely.

HERB-INFUSED BALMS

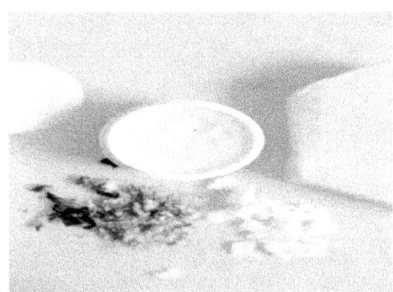

INGREDIENTS

Dry herbs

Carrier oil

Beeswax

Essential oils

RECOMMENDATIONS

Generate oils for 2-3 months in a tightly sealed box. Start again and you need to drop it if you discover mold growing.

Strain out the herbs

Combine oil and beeswax in saucepan or double boiler over low heat

When melted pour into clean containers and incorporate essential oils if desired

Let harden and salve cool

Shop in neat, dry place in lidded box.

Chickweed infused oil and salve

Ingredients:

Chickweed

Recipe Instructions: Herbal Oil Infusions: Chickweed oil may be used alone, or as a base for making chickweed salves and ointments

Coconut Oil Arnica Salve

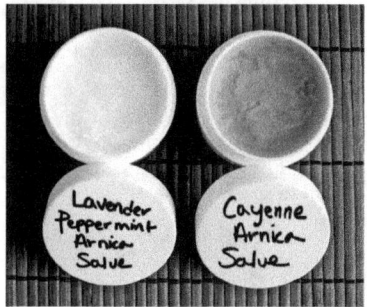

2 cups coconut oil

.6 ounces dried arnica montana flowers

¼ tsp. peppermint essential oil

½ cup beeswax granules

¼ tsp. lavender essential oil

Instructions:

1. Because you're using dry arnica, you will get best results if you can allow the arnica flowers to sharp in the coconut oil for 12-24 hours. I maintained my oven to the lowest setting possible and used a double boiler. Many people prefer a crock pot, and like this enables you to allow herbs large for an extended period of time.

2. Whiz it lightly in a food processor to begin bruising the flowers when you first get the arnica. You could also use your arms to crunch the plants up. This will enable the blossoms create the infusion of arnica happen a little faster and start to break down.

3. Place the dried arnica into crock pot or your double boiler. If you're making the cayenne salve, add the cayenne to the arnica as of this time.

4. Serve two glasses of coconut oil within the arnica and mix to make sure that all of the plants are fully submerged in the oil. You don't need any leaves sticking out.

5. Address and let impress on low temperature for 12-24 hours. You are able to stir it every so often if you desire. Watch about it to make sure the arnica all remains submerged and also to make sure that it doesn't get too hot.

6. Switch off the burner or crock pot when the given time has passed and allow the mixture cool for an hour. You don't want it to fully awesome, while the coconut oil might begin to solidify, but you want to buy to be cool enough that you don't burn yourself.

7. Place your cheesecloth, t-shirt, or pillowcase over container, your dish, or measuring cup. Carefully pour the coconut oil to the cheesecloth and allow the combination strain to the bowl below. If it's not too hot, you can grab the cheesecloth and press the oil through the material to speed up the method.

8. You can place the filtered oil back to your double boiler, once you've strained out the herbs. Be sure you wipe out the double boiler to make sure there are not any sections of herbs left in there. Turn the heat on low.

9. Add your beeswax and stir until completely dissolved. The short ½ cup of beeswax can deliver an incredibly soft salve. You can add more, if you want it firmer; softer, you can add less. You can test the feel by dropping the rear of a steel spoon into the combination and then allowing to great and using to your skin.

10. Once the beeswax is dissolved, remove from heat and let cool for about 30-60 minutes. Stir in your essential oils and then put into whatever containers you desire.

11. Utilize the salve on tired, aching muscles, bruises, injuries, arthritis, etc. NOTE: for the cayenne salve, use caution avoid applying to your face and when applying. If you're involved with pepper deposit on your fingers after implementing, you apply with a spool or small spatula, or may also use gloves. I personally use a spoon.

Lavender Chamomile Hand Salve

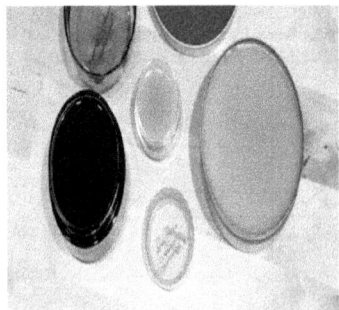

Ingredients

1/2 cup unrefined coconut oil

1/4 cup dried lavender

1/4 cup dried chamomile

2 Tbsp. beeswax

4-5 drops lavender essential oil

3-4 drops of any combination of tea tree, or orange, eucalyptus essential oils

Start by placing your coconut (or olive) oil in your saucepan on med-low heat. Add lavender and lavender. Stir to mix until hot. Lower heat and let it stay to impress for 20 minutes.

Secure cheesecloth over glass measuring cup with rubber bands.

Pour oil and flowers onto cheesecloth. Let oil drain into pot. After the plants are performed dripping and have cooled enough to manage, press extra oil from plants into pot. Be careful! Gas from the flowers may nevertheless be hot. Discard plants and the cheesecloth.

Rinse complete and saucepan with enough water to similar or exceed oil level in pot. Put on oven over spot and medium heat measuring cup in saucepan. Add beeswax to oil in measuring cup. Stir until wax is totally melted. Stir in essential oils and switch off heat.

Immediately pour into small, airtight containers for storage. Keep open and allow to cool completely before closing.

Chapter 4 – 15 Recipes

Burn Salve Recipe

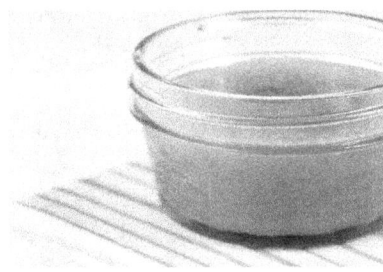

What You Need:

1/4 cup Raw Honey

1 Tablespoon Extra Virgin Coconut Oil

1 Tbsp Aloe Vera

Blow the mix together with a spoon if not with the electric hand machines. Shop in a little glass jar.

First clean the location with raw Apple Cider Vinegar when you need to use. This can help recover vitamins and vitamins to the skin and will also help restore the natural ph balance of the skin.

Apply the Burn Salve to the region, after washing the area with apple cider vinegar. So the burn can heal cover in gauze to retain the salve in a concentrated place. Of course, do not use this on burns that need medical attention.

Herbal Plantain Salve

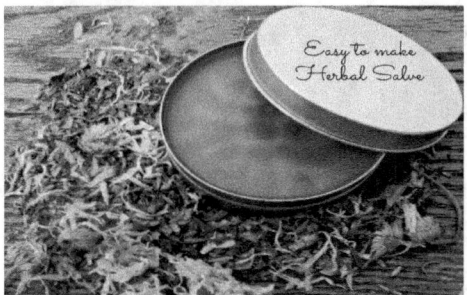

Instructions

Ensure your home equipment is DRY and clean. As water can cause your salve to form water and salve are not a great blend. 1. Have all the containers for pouring you want to complete available and ready.

1. Have all of the pots you wish to fill ready and available for serving. This may make it easier than fumbling around when everything is dissolved.

2. Evaluate beeswax and your infused oil and put into small pot. Heat over low, stirring before wax is melted. Remove from heat.

3. Add 5 drops of E Vitamin oil and 5 drops of grapefruit seed extract and mix. I add a fall for every ounce of oil and wax, the grapefruit seed extract and E Vitamin may behave as preservatives for your salve.

4. If you are going to include essential oils, now's the time. I love the smell of rose and it has its own healing properties which might be excellent for skin and wound care. A shed or two of peppermint taste and smell wonderful if you plan on using your salve for chap stick.

5. Serve the warmed oil mixture into a glass measuring cup that has a pourable spout. This makes putting into pots so much easier. Work with a rubber spatula to get the oil in the attributes of the container.

6. Carefully fill your oil in your package(s) of choice. The salve will begin to harden up quickly so you need to go as fast as you can without dropping.

Capsaicin Cream Recipe

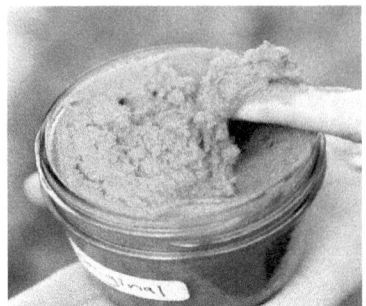

You will need...

-3 tablespoons of cayenne powder

-1 cup of grapeseed oil

-1/2 cup of grated beeswax

-A double boiler

-A glass jar with a tightly fitting lid

Directions

Mix together 3 tablespoons of cayenne powder with 1 cup of your oil of choice and heat in a double boiler for 5-10 minutes over medium heat. Stir in a 1/2 pot of grated beeswax and continue to mix until it has melted completely and everything is mixed together. Chill the combination in the freezer for 10 minutes, and then whisk together. Chill for another 10-15 and then beat again before putting it in a glass bottle with a closely fitting lid and storing in the refrigerator. It'll keep for 1 ½ months-use daily as required for pain.

Super-Strength Cream

The hotter the pepper, the more capsaicin it has, making this product super strength.

You'll need...

-1 cup of beeswax

-4 tablespoons of Habanero powder

-4 cups of grapeseed or another oil, including olive, jojoba, or almond

-Gloves

-A double boiler

-A glass jar with a tightly fitting lid

Directions

Mix 4 tablespoons of Habanero powder with 4 servings of grapeseed or olive oil in a double boiler. Let this mix warm up over medium heat for 5-10 minutes. Melt 1 cup of beeswax in to the mixture after it's warmed till everything is smoothly blended together and mix it. Allow it to relax for 10 minutes in the freezer and whisk. Chill for another 10-15 minutes and then beat together once more before refrigerating it and pouring into a glass container with a tightly fitting lid. It will retain its efficiency for 1 1/2 days. Apply as needed for pain, preventing use if any irritation occurs.

Little Bit Extra Cream

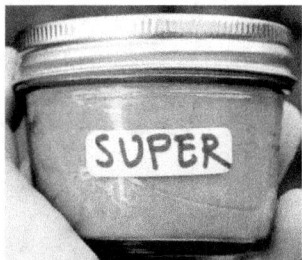

This treatment involves one other notable anti- inflammatory and pain reducers turmeric and cinnamon, in addition to cayenne.

You'll need...

-3 cups of grapeseed oil, or any other oil like almond, jojoba, or olive

-3 tablespoons of ground cayenne

-1/2 cup of beeswax

-3 tablespoons of turmeric

-2 tablespoons of ground ginger

-A double boiler

Directions

Mix together 3 tablespoons of ground cayenne, 3 tablespoons of turmeric, and 2 tablespoons of ground cinnamon. Add this to 3 servings of grapeseed oil in a double boiler and stir until blended thoroughly. Hot medium heat for 5-10 minutes over and adding in 1/2 cup of beeswax. Stir until the beeswax has melted completely and everything is blended together, and then remove from heat and chill in the refrigerator for 10 minutes. After 10 minutes mixing it yet again by the end and whisk it together and then refrigerate for another 10, take it out. Place in a glass bottle with a closely fitting lid in the refrigerator, where it'll retain for 1 ½ months. Apply then let it dry before rinsing off and as required for pain, but with this treatment, wipe in up to you can. The turmeric can really mark.

When you use your cream, definitely take the time to gently rub it into each tender joint. The little bit of pleasure helps get your circulation pumping and moves body through your bones. This gets vitamins to them and oxygen, that will be particularly good for osteoarthritis. Don't forget to wear gloves when controlling very hot stuff and stop using if it causes a lot of discomfort.

Rub For Sore Muscles Recipes

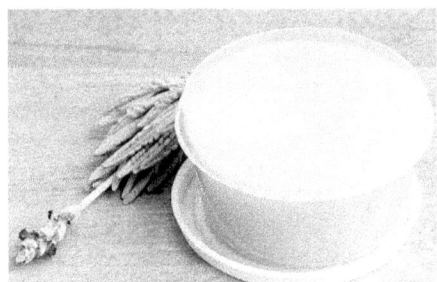

What You'll Need:

Small saucepan

Small heat-safe bowl

1/4 cup coconut oil

1/4 cup olive oil

1 tablespoon beeswax

1/4 teaspoon ground pepper

1/4 teaspoon ground ginger

20 drops peppermint essential oil

20 drops eucalyptus essential oil

20 drops clove oil

Directions:

Start with answering a little pot with water and locating a heatproof dish that may fit inside the pot. You can even use a clean may for this task. Measure and include the olive and coconut oil to the bowl, along with the ground pepper and cinnamon. Deliver the water to a simmer, and then allow the mix warm in the hot water for 20 minutes.

Black pepper and cinnamon are more than just herbs! Support and ingredients are warming with flow, soothing sore muscles. After 20 minutes of steeping in the oils, add the beeswax, and heat until melted.

Place a strainer over a little bowl, and add a bit of extra help with a coffee filter. Remove in the pot, and pour over the strainer. This keeps the cinnamon and ground pepper out of your smooth salve.

Now add eucalyptus essential oils and the peppermint. Both smell fresh and invigorating and add a deep, soothing tingle to the stroke.

Carefully fill the heating stroke in a little sealable container, and let set at room temperature for a pair of hours. Top, and use when your muscles are in need of some comforting.

Dandelion Salve Recipe

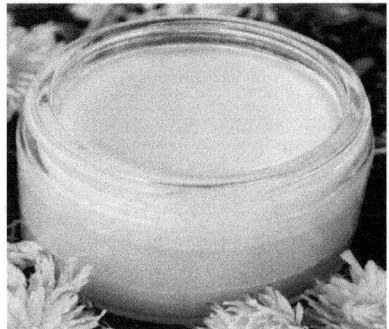

We first need to create an infused oil to make our salve. The problem with using recently picked dandelions for this is they've this type of high water content, that your oil can get a little sludgy and major sometimes, with a higher probability of spoilage.

The size of the vessel is determined by how many dandelions you have. To get a small amount of dandelions, use a small jar; if your supply is big, use a bigger jar. Don't get hung on correct numbers and amounts. You're basically filling some type of package about 1/2 to 3/4 whole with wilted dandelion plants then addressing them with oil.

Set gently into a pot of heated water and heat gradually over medium low heat. Allow the oil stay in the heated water for a long time remove.

Now, you can proceed and stress the oil and use in your salve or you could allow it impress several days longer in a black cabinet. Another option is to stress the oil then do the whole process again with freshly wilted flowers and the initial set of dandelion oil. It is a double infusion.

This makes an excellent massage oil. It's especially nice if you add in a few drops of soothing lavender essential oil.

Once our oil is finished infusing, we're ready to create some salve!

Homemade Bloodroot Salve

1) Grind the roots, sometimes together or independently, with care not to heat them past 100 degrees Fahrenheit. But don't work them until needed, keeping them closed and dried to guard strength.

2) Set the zinc chloride in an open glass bowl. Add a little amount of distilled water for simplicity in blending, if needed.

3) Slowly mix the roots in to the zinc, utilizing a wooden spoon, stir thoroughly.

The zinc may heat since it oxidizes, slightly cooking the roots, allowing the alkaloids mixture and to release to the option.

Permit it to liquefy (oxidize) uncovered. In a humid and warm weather, zinc chloride may liquefy faster. In dry and cold climates, it might take up to 5 days. The method wills hasten. Try not to add water if you don't need the medicine quickly. It works best if made to resemble the consistency of toothpaste.

4) Check the pH of the mixture, it should range between 3.7 and 3.8. Add more powdered root, in equal measure, to accomplish this array, serving also the thicken the mixture.

5) Place small portions of the finished combination in small glass or cosmetic-type jars. These jars should hide seal and light air completely. Never use metal containers or items.

6) We recommend the Salve be refrigerated if held for long-term storage, particularly in hot climates.

Bloodroot salve, also known as drawing salve, can be a corrosive herbal substance that is applied to skin over tumors, skin tags, moles and infections.

The original Native American variety of Salve was really created from blood root and crushed wood ash, and perhaps bone ash too. More modern evolutions tend to be different, work differently as.

Other common ingredients include:

chaparral

chickweed

Indian tobacco

comfrey

myrrh

marshmallow

mullein

Sodom's apple

Olive oil. Some choose to include oil like a load, particularly in the event of parasites or heavy rashes.

Black Drawing Salve Recipe

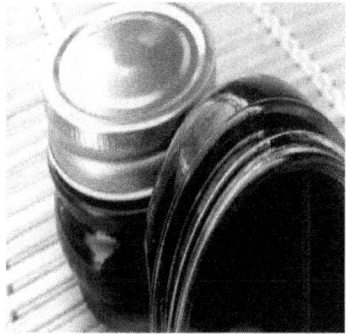

Ingredients

3 comfrey Tablespoons

2 teaspoons shea butter

2 Tablespoons coconut oil

2 Tablespoons Beeswax

1 teaspoon Vitamin E oil

2 Tablespoons Activated Charcoal Powder

2 Tablespoons Kaolin Clay

1 Tablespoon honey

20 drops Lavender Gas

Instructions

It is crucial to generate olive oil with calendula, comfrey and plantain before making the salve. You ½ cup olive oil, finely powdered in blender or a food processor, and will need 1 tablespoon of each of the herbs. It can be infused in one of those two ways:

Dust place and the herbs in a small jar. Pour within the herbs. Leave in vessel for 3-4 days, moving daily, and then strain via a cheesecloth for use.

Heat the herbs and olive oil in a double boiler. Keep on low/medium heat for about one hour until oil gets deeper and strong smell. Strain through cheesecloth for use.

Personally, I keep a big jar of olive oil with plantain, comfrey and calendula in my plant cabinet and allow it to constantly infuse for use in salves and lotions. I discard the herbs and start the process again when the oil can be used.

Mix infused olive oil, shea butter, coconut oil, beeswax, Vitamine oil and baby in a glass jar in a small pot of water.

Heat the water to a simmer and carefully stir mixture in the vessel until all ingredients are dissolved.

Remove from heat and include lavender essential oil, kaolin clay, and activated charcoal and mix well.

Quickly fill in to small jars or cans and let remain until hardened (several hours).

Shop in airtight container and use as needed on cuts, splinters, etc.

Salve for Cracked Heels

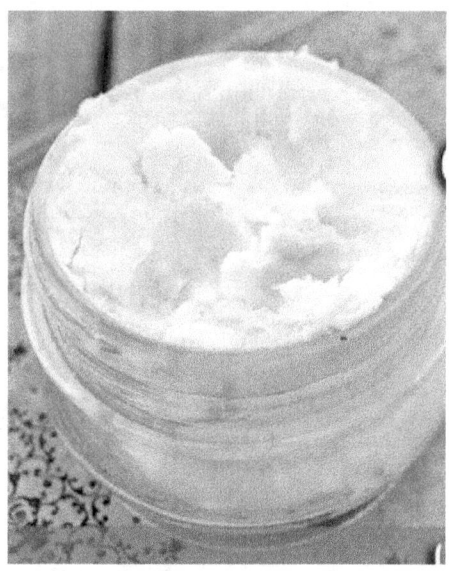

Cracked Heel Foot Salve Ingredients

¼ cup Coconut Oil

¼ cup Shea Butter

3 Beeswax Tablespoons

¼ cup Magnesium Flakes + 2 Tablespoons boiling water

10 drops Oregano Essential Oil

10 drops Peppermint Essential Oil

What to Do:

Put 2 tablespoons of boiling water in to the magnesium flakes in a small container and stir until it dissolves. This can produce a thick liquid. Reserve to cool.

In a quart size mason jar inside a little pot with 1-inch of water, combine the coconut oil, beeswax and shea butter and switch on medium heat.

Take away the jar from the pan, when dissolved and allow mix slightly opaque and cool until room temperature. At this point, put in to a medium bowl or in to a blender.

If in a jar, utilize immersion blender or a hand blender on medium-speed and start joining the oil mixture.

Slowly (starting with a decline at a time) incorporate the dissolved magnesium blend to the oil mixture while continuous blending until all of the magnesium combination is included and it's well-mixed.

Include the oregano and peppermint essential oils if using and beat until combined.

Set in the refrigerator for fifteen minutes and re-blend to get body butter consistency.

Store in refrigerator for a cooling cream or at room temperature for up to 8 weeks.

Use on cracked heels at night. Implement a thick layer and wear socks before salve absorbs. For best results, exfoliate feet with dry skin using Ped Egg or the pumice, then execute a detoxifying foot soak, let dry and use the salve. Repeat as needed until problem resolves.

Pregnancy Stretch Marks Salve

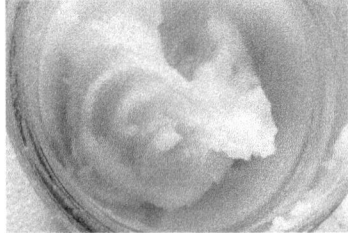

Stretchmarks Salve Ingredients

1/4 cup Shea Butter

1/4 cup coconut oil

3 Tablespoons Apricot Kernel Oil

1 Tablespoon Calendula flowers (optional)

1/4 teaspoon dried ginger root

How to Make Stretch Marks Salve

Dry ginger and if using the calendula, add to Almond Oil or Apricot-Kernel and location in pan or a double boiler over a small pan of water. (or utilize a glass vessel for easier tidy up)

Provide to a simmer and warmth for 30 minutes on medium-low temperature to combine the properties of the herbs.

Stress through metal or a cheesecloth strainer to remove herbs. You'll want to ensure you still have at least 2 tablespoons of liquid oil left.

Return the oil to the double boiler and include coconut oil and the shea butter.

Temperature until melted and stir to combine.

Remove from store and heat in small glass jar.

Include any pregnancy-safe essential oils if desired.

Use as needed on skin before, during or after pregnancy as needed.

Healing Lip Salve Recipe

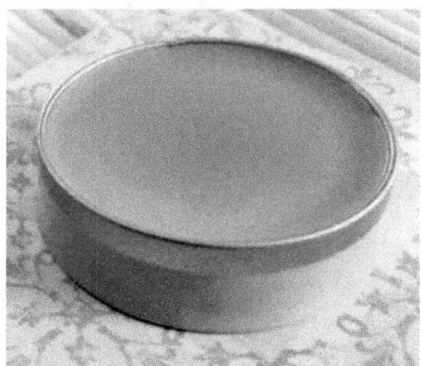

Lip Balm Ingredients

1 cup of olive or almond oil

1 teaspoon echinacea root

1 teaspoon comfrey leaf

1 teaspoon plantain leaf

1 teaspoon calendula flowers

1 teaspoon yarrow flowers

1 teaspoon rosemary leaf

1/4 cup beeswax pastilles

grapefruit seed extract or vitamin E oil

peppermint essential oil

5-10 drops of peppermint essential oil

Lip Balm Instructions

Generate the herbs to the olive oil. There are two ways to try this. You can either combine the herbs and the olive oil in a container with an airtight lid and keep 3-4 months, moving daily OR heat the herbs and olive oil over low/low heat in a double boiler for 3 hours before oil is quite natural. You can also abandon this task entirely, or simply a decrease of each of the essential oils instead.

Stress the herbs out of the oil by flowing through a cheesecloth. Allow all the oil spill out and then fit the herbs to get out the residual oil.

Discard the herbs.

Temperature 1/4 glass of the infused oil in a double boiler with the beeswax until melted and mixed.

Pour into tiny tins, glass containers or top chap tubes and use on dry or chapped lips.

CALENDULA - COMFREY SALVE RECIPE

Here is some things you'll need:

1 cup of organic, cold pressed olive oil

1-ounce total of dried plant - in this event 1/2 oz of calendula and 1/2 ounce of comfrey

1/2 ounce of grated beeswax

3 vitamin E capsules that is your chemical

Cheesecloth to strain herbs

Let's get started!

Place your herbs into an oven safe dish and serve the olive oil in. Stir and cook in the range at the lowest possible temperature and make for 3 hours. This is called an herbal infused oil.

After 3 hours permit the mix to cool slightly but strain through the cheesecloth although it is still warm. Make sure to fit out every one of the oil you can.

Now put your mixture in a box to the stove and very LIGHTLY heat the oil blend back up. DO NOT BURN IT!

Hole and add your vitamin E supplements and adding your beeswax. Stir until it is totally melted and mixed.

Remove from heat and let cool merely a second or two then put into a wide mouth jar or several small jars. As it cools the mix will end up semisolid and the ideal salve consistency!

Cansema Black Salve Recipe # 1

One tablespoon each powdered bloodroot and polk root

1 tablespoon zinc chloride

One tablespoon Charcoal

Vitamin A, 10,000 IU

Wood tar

Pascalite clay

Reduce the zinc chloride in one to two tablespoons of warm distilled water. Use only enough water to dissolve. Set aside.

Mix bloodroot, polk and charcoal root in a different box with a little cooking oil, just enough to protect the herbs, mix well. Carefully add the zinc chloride and water mix, stirring well. Gently heat the mix in double boiler, stirring continuously for 30 minuets Remove from heat, mix well, let cool, add DMSO.

Next, mix one teaspoon to one tablespoon in a time of the Pascalite clay to the bloodroot mix until you've a clean, thick paste that is easily spreadable. Do not put of the clay in to the mixture or it'll be uneven. When the combination is too dense, add a few drops of oil or water to thin. If thin, add a touch more of the clay. The clay is important in this formula as it helps to remove impurities in the skin. If you do not have clay and need to produce the paste instantly, it may be thickened with flour.

You'll only need to implement this substance once. Use to the cancer, address with gauze and recording (bandaids will not function), leave undisturbed for 12 hours. At the end of 12 hours, wash area with soap and water, and then clean with hydrogen peroxide. This is applied every 2-3 days if you feel you need to, generally one software is all that is required for tiny cancers. The cancer may disappear by itself in one to five months. Your might have burning or pain, fever, stinging, extreme irritation; this is normal. You may employ some chickweed salve to the area for the irritation, but don't use anything else including healing salves. The area wills heal up before it has time to eliminate the cancer.

Cansema Black Salve Recipe # 2

Cansema is a natural skin cancer treatment. Cansema's active ingredients are Zinc, bloodroot, and chaparral. It may be obtained from Alpha Omega Labs in the Bahamas. There's a Recipe available.

This can be a menu for a dark paste very similar to the Cansema. But it is a favorite substance for cancer and all suspect skin cancer like lesions. This paste also has worked well for all manner of cancers so long as they've become exposed to or close to the top of your skin.

1/2 cup powdered Blood Root

1/2 cup Zinc Chloride, crystals or liquid

1/2 cup common white flour

1 1/2 cup hot water

Pre-mix before adding to the water all but the water, completely. Boiler doubles. Put in water, then mix in the other ingredients. Stir in nicely employing a wooden spoon. Cook for 30 mins over boiling water, stirring constantly. Request is a lot exactly like Cansema. Apply a thin layer (2-3mm) of the stick within the affected region and address for 24 hours. Then eliminate the masking but don't disrupt the patch at all, don't attempt to pull out the cancer at any time, it will fall out in 10 days. Many people with delicate skin put Vaseline round the cancer so the stick does not irritate your skin.

Conclusion

What Are Herbal Salves & Creams?

An herbal salve is just a blend of herbal infused oils that are thickened with some kind of wax (most commonly beeswax) such that it will be in a great form at room temperature.

An herbal cream is quite similar. It begins as a salve but is shaped in to a product by blending a water in to the oils with the support of an emulsifier to maintain both opposites from separating. Products may differ in color along with in persistence, but most are off-white and soft.

How Do Creams & Salves Work?

For that most part, creams and salves work locally, meaning their outcomes are reserved for wherever you use them. They're not going to act systemically like specific topical medications will. I'm not saying they can't. The skin is just a complex organ that's extremely absorbent, but it's also extremely particular as to what it permits to make it through its sheets and to the system.

There's a whole process that topical products have to undergo in order for their chemicals to get to the bloodstream. What makes it to the system is nowhere near to what was actually put on the top of your skin. I recently stumbled on this post over at Herb & Hedgerow that does an excellent job considering this matter of the skin's power to absorb, just how much it absorbs, whether it absorbs everything placed on it or not, and what really makes it to the blood stream. It's really interesting, and if you're interested in learning more about toxins and I'd highly suggest reading it, why it's recommended to use natural products as a portion of your skincare routine.

Because herbal salves are primarily made up of oil and wax, it take longer to enter the sheets of your skin and will lay on top of the skin. Which means the herbal properties take longer to get in to the skin's cells. An herbal cream around the other hand may enter the skin's sheets more quickly because it contains water. This will help to hold the herbal properties deeper in the areas at a faster pace compared to the salve would.

If you need the preparation to enter quickly your best choice is to:

Utilize a treatment or some preparation that contains water

Massage the region or use heat to ensure that blood flow to those tissues are increased.

All of these things may help to enter the skin faster therefore taking the herbal properties into the areas more quickly.

Now, please know that I'm in no techniques saying a product is preferable to a salve as it gets to the cells faster. Sometimes you need these properties to last longer, however there are other occasions when you may want faster reduction. Actually, there's not much room to mess up here. Both products support to get the herbal properties into the skin.

When To NOT Use Salves & Creams On The Skin

Like I said earlier, for properties to be absorbed into the system to allow them to have an effect on the whole body or if you're searching for deep penetration, salves and products aren't your best solution. Herbal powders, tinctures, teas, and liniments look to become more appropriate.

Another time when you wouldn't need to use even a product or a salve about the skin is if you've broken even a deep wound or skin. Sure, scraps and cuts are thought broken skin and a thin layer of an antibacterial salve is definitely correct for that, but I'm talking about pieces that need stitches or big gaping wounds from the dog bite or something similar. Salves and creams are likely to stop air so its superior to use herbal washes and/or herbal oils in the place of arrangements that have waxes from capture bacteria in serious wounds and getting to the cells.

Think About Preservation?

When you create something from scratch, over time, yeast, bacteria, and form can grow, particularly in products which contain water. So when it comes to increasing the shelf life of your products and keeping gross issues from increasing in them, you've two options.

Salt

Natural Preservatives

Salt come in numerous varieties and are based on the products pH along with the kind of preparation you need to preserve. Products are partially preserved by some while others fully maintain the merchandise. While some don't some contain parabens and formaldehyde, and virtually all of them are synthetic.

Organic additives about the other hand are protected, however they don't sustain a product the way preservative chemicals do. This implies you need to take a few extra measures to discourage bacteria, yeast, and form from developing in what you make.

Keep things clean... very clean, before and through the process. That is essentially the most important step you usually take in preventing contamination.

So you use them quickly make things in small pockets, and be sure to store them properly. Water, heat, and light are three things that can compromise products and develop an environment where gross things can grow.

Use natural preservatives to decrease gross items from rising rapidly.

Now, some individuals who create skincare products can stress the significance of preserving your products; however, there are several of us who've just applied natural preservatives with great success. In my head, if you don't wish to use substances in your products, you can find things you can perform to expand your shelf life and keep your products safe for those using them. You might not be able to mass- let them sit in a warehouse or on store shelves for weeks at a time, but who would like to fit old products on their body anyway and produce your items. I'm all for new and natural whenever possible! Does more research with this subject to find out about what you may do?

Pure maintenance is something I examine in greater detail in the e book below. It's a must-examine if you wish to know more about this topic without doing all of the research yourself!

How To Make An Herbal Salve

Now for the fun part. Action-by-step instructions on how to make your own herbal salve.

Once your herbal infused oil is finished and strained, dissolve wax in a small saucepan. The standard rate for oil to feel is 1-ounce of wax for every cup of oil. Of course this may vary dependent on how hard you need your salve to end up, but that's the overall rule of thumb.

Once your wax is melted, convert off heat and add your herbal infused oil to the wax. Stir well.

Bottle in tins or glass jars. Brand and store.

How To Make An Herbal Cream

To create an herbal treatment, you're going to follow the steps above for making a salve with just a few versions.

Decide what fluid you're going to use in your treatment, before infusing your herbs into your oil. Water? Hydrosol? Aloe solution or juice? Let this fluid sit out about the table so that it can come to room temperature while you work through the rest of the actions.

Follow the steps above for creating an herbal salve just don't jar the salve up when it's completed. Keep it in the saucepan to cool. Since the salve cools it'll begin to thicken.

Once your salve has thickened but is very gentle and still warm, use a plastic spatula to discard the edges of the saucepan and combine the salve well.

Next having an immersion blender, slowly combine the salve on low-speed while slowly putting in the water you chose. The proportion of salve to fluid for a cream is usually 50:50. If you have 1 cup of salve, then you'll blend in 1 cup of water. This may vary based on how solid or thin you want your product to be. It's also important the salve and water be as close to each other in temperature as possible for the emulsion to occur. If one's too warm and the other's too cool, the oil and water may not mix at all or may separate later.

Once the fluid and the salve continues to be mixed together nicely and you will find fluids or no salve sections growing to the top of your cream, you're all completed. Just put into store, and glass jars or cans, brand. Know that more will thicken since it continues to cool.